NATURAL REMEDIES

by
Christopher Day MA, VetMB, MRCVS, VetFFHom

Illustrations by
Carole Vincer

KENILWORTH PRESS

First published in Great Britain by
The Kenilworth Press Limited,
Addington, Buckingham, MK18 2JR

© The Kenilworth Press Limited 1996
Reprinted 1997

British Library Cataloguing in Publication Data
A catalogue record for this book is available from the British Library.

ISBN 1-872082-79-3

Typeset by The Kenilworth Press Limited

Printed in Great Britain by Westway Offset, Wembley

My thanks to Caroline Beaney for typing the manuscript

The law: legislation relevant to this booklet
Veterinary Surgeons Act, 1966; Medicines Act, 1968; Cruelty to Animals Act, 1911

The implication of this legislation is that it is only a qualified veterinary surgeon who may legally treat or prescribe for your horse. There are many non-veterinarians who set out to treat horses but it is an unfortunate sequel to the Veterinary Surgeons Act that, if an owner consults a non-vet and thereby fails to alleviate suffering for his or her animal, prosecution under the 1911 Act is a possibility.
 It is also worthwhile to study Food Labelling Legislation, which will aid in the understanding of the declared ingredients on horse feed and supplement labels.

CONTENTS

NATURAL REMEDIES

4 Introduction
5 Nutrition and diet
6 Shoeing and saddlery
7 Homœopathy
8 Herbs
9 Other natural therapies
10 Injuries and first aid
12 Abscess
12 Allergy
13 Arthritis
14 Back problems
15 Colic
15 Cough
16 Diarrhœa
16 Discharges
17 Feet
19 Laminitis
19 Mud fever/Greasy heel
20 Nervousness and excitability
20 Ringworm
21 Saddle sores
21 Splint
22 Sprained tendons, ligaments and muscles
23 Sweet itch
23 Windgalls
24 Guide to dosing and administration

Introduction ■ ■ ■ ■ ■ ■ ■ ■ ■ ■ ■ ■ ■ ■ ■ ■

The modern horse lives a life far removed from that of his ancestors. Domestication imposes unnatural living conditions and also usually requires the horse to perform some kind of work. Sadly these factors can lead to disease rather more often than we would like.

This book sets out not only to help mitigate the possible harmful effects of modern lifestyle, nutrition and work but also to suggest easy natural remedies for many of the common ailments to which a horse may fall prey.

It is intended that those who care for horses should be able, in many cases, to treat common ailments themselves both promptly and effectively, thus ensuring the greatest chance of rapid recovery. They should be able to recognise disease and administer natural medication according to their own particular expertise or leaning. For this reason this book lays out information on different forms of natural therapy, including homœopathy, herbs, tissue salts, Bach Flower remedies, essential oils etc. It also gives a brief description of these forms of therapy. Acupuncture is excluded as it is not do-it-yourself medicine.

Nutrition and diet are the key to good health and for this reason there is a section devoted to this most fundamentally important area. While natural medicine provides a stimulus to healing, a healthy diet is essential to health and will speed recovery.

The book is directed at caring horse riders or keepers who wish to take some degree of responsibility for their charges. It is not intended to be a substitute for veterinary surgeons, whose help should always be sought in cases of serious illness. However, be warned, as yet there are extremely few veterinarians who treat horses in the way this book describes.

Nutrition and Diet

The modern domesticated horse has evolved over an estimated 45 million years from a small, dog-sized creature browsing in rich vegetation and forests in the Eocene epoch to a large, fast running, powerful, plains-dwelling creature who feeds mainly on grass, herbs and fibrous plant material in present times.

His teeth and digestive system have developed to handle roughage. The teeth are a very powerful milling device, breaking up stemmy material before it passes into the stomach. Food eventually finds its way into the large intestine which acts as a huge fermentation vat, breaking it down into smaller and smaller components with the help of bacteria and other micro-organisms.

A horse should be fed a natural diet, as close to his evolved needs as possible. Avoid unsuitable by-products, artificial vitamins, beet pulp, molasses and sugar by-products, chemical antioxidants and other preservatives, etc., which may disturb normal function of the bowel flora upon which the horse depends. Supplements are rarely necessary and should follow the above principles. They should be properly integrated and compatible with the main diet so as not to create imbalances.

The best basic diet for a horse is grass from traditional pasture containing a wealth of plant species, or hay from similar ground. Artificial fertilisers should be avoided. If extra feed is necessary, stick to unadulterated raw materials, such as oats, barley, bran, etc.

If organic food is obtained, so much the better. A great deal of disease, both of the mind and of the body, can be strongly influenced by diet. No medicine is complete without dietary support, so dietary work should be integral with medicine.

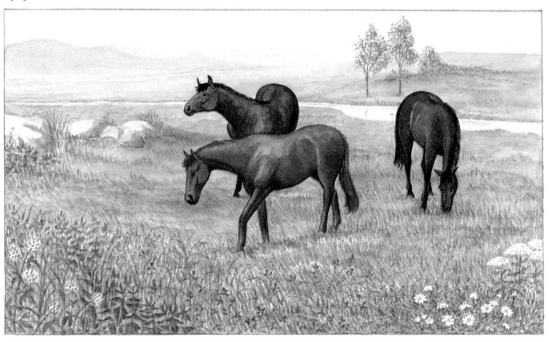

Shoeing and Saddlery

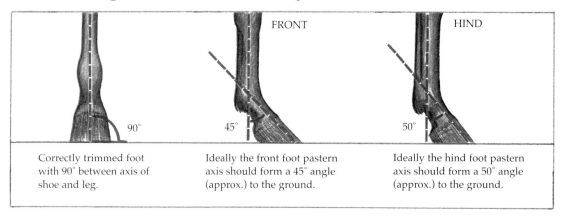

FRONT   HIND

90°   45°   50°

Correctly trimmed foot with 90° between axis of shoe and leg.	Ideally the front foot pastern axis should form a 45° angle (approx.) to the ground.	Ideally the hind foot pastern axis should form a 50° angle (approx.) to the ground.

The saddles or harness put on the horse's back and the metal shoes applied to his feet can, in conjunction with the way he is worked, exert a decisive effect on his health.

A horse's leg is built for fore and aft movement, not sideways movement. The shape of his foot, both in respect of toe length in relation to heel length, and in respect of the side-to-side balance of the foot, is therefore vital. Feet should be trimmed and shoes applied such that a horse's foot always lands flat when his leg is used vertically (i.e. there should be 90° between the axis of the shoe and the axis of the leg when viewed from the front).

The saddle should be fitted so that the seat proper is horizontal when the saddle is placed in the correct position on the horse's back (i.e. far enough back to allow free movement of the shoulder). The saddle should be central on the back when viewed from behind with the horse standing square. The tree at the pommel should be wide enough to allow the muscles of the wither to function. The pommel should have sufficient clearance over the top of the wither. The seat and cantle should not bounce on the horse's back during work. Apart from this, all other tack should fit properly, be comfortable and should be maintained in tip-top condition.

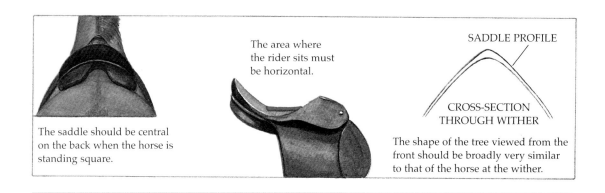

The saddle should be central on the back when the horse is standing square.

The area where the rider sits must be horizontal.

SADDLE PROFILE

CROSS-SECTION THROUGH WITHER

The shape of the tree viewed from the front should be broadly very similar to that of the horse at the wither.

Homœopathy

Homœopathy is a system of medicine using the extracts of plants, minerals and some animal material (usually diluted to an extreme extent) to cure disease by the law of similars. This law was discovered by Samuel Hahnemann in Germany in 1790 when he found that a substance could cure a disease syndrome if it was able to produce broadly similar symptoms in a healthy body.

Plant material, for instance, is usually made into a remedy by extraction in alcohol, followed by filtering and serial dilution, commonly to six or thirty stages each of 1/100, with succussion (violent shaking) at each stage. These would be labelled 6c and 30c respectively. The 6c is more readily obtainable.

The medicines are safe, gentle and free of side-effects, can be given to pregnant or suckling mares and are an extremely powerful stimulus to healing when properly used.

Storage of remedies in a cool, even temperature in glass bottles in the dark is a very valuable precaution, in order to preserve their efficacy. Strong-smelling substances should not be stored near them.

Homœopathic remedies can be purchased as tablets, pillules, powders, crystals or liquids. Any of these, to suit the reader's preferences, should be given by mouth to the horse, making sure not to touch the material by hand en route, as this will tend to destroy the remedy's efficacy. **It should not be given with a meal of concentrate feed.**

Dose rates do not vary with the size of the horse. For convenience the author suggests 4 tablets, 6 pillules, a half teaspoon of powder, or 10 drops of liquid remedies as a dose, depending upon the form in which the remedy is purchased.

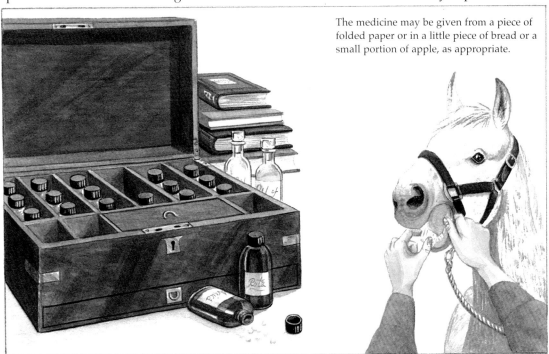

The medicine may be given from a piece of folded paper or in a little piece of bread or a small portion of apple, as appropriate.

Herbs

Horses respond well to herbal medicine and many believe that a horse in the wild is able to select his own plant medicine, given adequate choice of growing herbs. This is difficult to prove, but certainly the horse is a very intuitive and sensitive creature. For this reason alone, it is very unwise to follow the modern route of 'pasture improvement', reducing the number of available species to a minimum and artificially fertilising the ground, thus destroying indefinitely its natural mineral and organic balance.

Each herb is a complex collection of mineral and organic material, some of whose ingredients are clearly discernible, medically active compounds. They exist as part of the whole and constitute a valuable medicine together, each ingredient playing a part in the balance. Avoid single extracts where an ingredient has been isolated from its holistic, whole-herb context.

Herbs are grouped into several categories, according to their general effect on the body or its tissues and organs. Some of these categories are **Alteratives** (which gradually restore proper function to the body), **Astringents** (which tend to dry secretions and discharges), **Bitters** (which stimulate the stomach), **Demulcents** (which soothe inflamed internal tissues), **Emollients** (which soothe inflamed external tissues), and **Vulneraries** (which treat injuries).

These can be used singly or multiply, in order to achieve the desired medicinal effect and balance. There is an art to selecting and mixing herbs to achieve a proper balanced effect. Herbs may be used in conjunction with other forms of therapy.

Dose rates of individual herbs vary and can be very important. By and large,

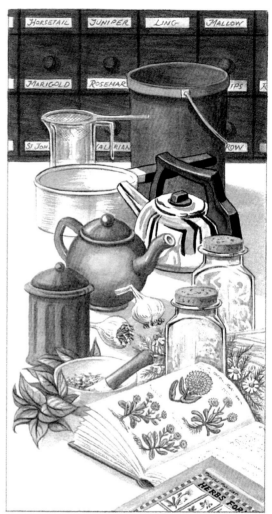

the herbs mentioned in the text are less dose-sensitive but doses often range between 5 and 30 grams of dried material.

Beware products marketed by those with no tradition, experience or knowledge of herbal medicine. Some herbs can be dangerous, particularly if dosed regularly.

Comfrey has, in my opinion, received some unjustified bad press lately, but I have used it without mishap and find it a very valuable remedy.

Other Natural Therapies

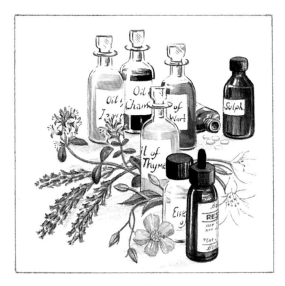

Bach Flowers

Edward Bach devised this very intuitive system of natural medicine in the 1930s. He harnessed the curative energy of flowers, mostly by steeping them in an alcohol/water mixture and exposing them to strong sunlight. The Bach Flowers act on medical problems via the mental aspects of disease and are selected mostly via a study of psychological/ behavioural clues. They can have a powerful effect and this is most clearly to be seen in the combination preparation, Rescue Remedy, which is used in emergency and stress situations. Its calming and curative effects can be extraordinary. There are, in all, thirty-eight remedies. Ten drops will count as a dose, given by mouth.

Tissue salts

In the nineteenth century, Dr Schuessler formulated a hypothesis and demonstrated that medical problems stemmed from a biochemical imbalance centred on the exchange of mineral salts both in the cells and in extracellular fluids. Twelve salts are used, either singly or in combination, to rebalance the body and they are obtainable in low potencies, prepared in a similar way to homoeopathic medicines. The 'potency' is usually 6x. These medicines should be treated carefully just like homoeopathic medicines and should be given by mouth. They come as tablets.

Essential oils

These oils have for thousands of years been extracted from plants and used as very powerful medicinal substances. They may be used as massages or as inhalations and represent a diverse and versatile medical tool. Their use is inevitably related to herbal medicine but deserves special mention, since they contain a different combination of ingredients from their parent herbs and operate differently. Within limits they are safe to use but caution is needed with some, especially during pregnancy.

When massaging, take care not to blister the skin with oils which are too strong or to massage too vigorously or for too long.

Magnet therapy

Relatively new on the market are small magnets which can be applied to local injuries, thus exploiting the healing properties of the magnetic field.

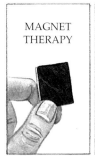
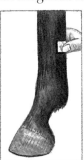
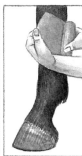

MAGNET THERAPY

Injuries and First aid

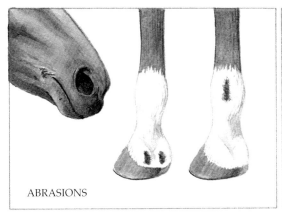

ABRASIONS

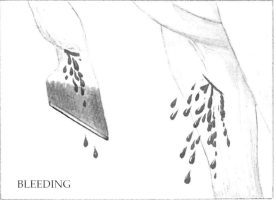

BLEEDING

In all cases of injury, assessment must be made as to whether veterinary help is needed. Even if it is, then a few appropriate first-aid measures, applied promptly, can limit the damage caused by injury and can speed healing. (For instance, prompt and consistent homœopathic help will usually prevent totally the problem of proud flesh in wounds and wound infection.)

If the horse is shocked
* *Homœopathy:* **Aconite**
* *Bach Flowers:* **Rescue Remedy**
* *Essential oils:* **Camphor** or **Melissa** (by inhalation)

If there are abrasions
* *Homœopathy:* Topical **Hypericum and Calendula** lotion, diluted 1 in 10

If there is a bruise
* *Homœopathy:* **Arnica** internally, **Arnica lotion** externally
* *Essential oils:* **Hyssop** (gentle massage)

If there is a cut wound
* *Homœopathy:* **Staphysagria** and topical **Hypericum and Calendula** lotion, diluted 1 in 10

If there is bony injury
* *Homœopathy:* **Symphytum, Arnica**
* *Herbs:* **Comfrey**

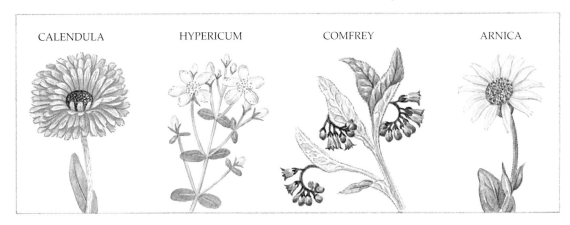

CALENDULA   HYPERICUM   COMFREY   ARNICA

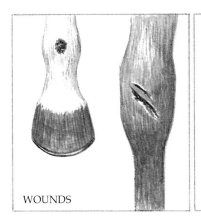

WOUNDS

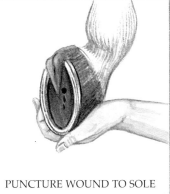

PUNCTURE WOUND TO SOLE

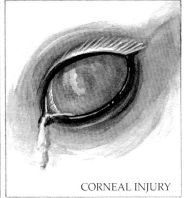

CORNEAL INJURY

If there is a puncture/stab wound
(e.g. nail; NB: Danger of tetanus)
- *Homœopathy:* **Ledum** and topical **Hypericum and Calendula** lotion, diluted 1 in 10
If it is in the hoof, first open the wound carefully to allow drainage (see Abscess).

If there is a sprain
- *Homœopathy:* **Ruta**
- *Herbs:* **Comfrey**
- *Essential oils:* **Eucalyptus**, **Lavender** and **Rosemary** (massage)

If there is oedema
- *Homœopathy:* **Apis mel.**
- *Tissue salts:* **Nat. mur., Nat. sulph.**

If there is haemorrhage
- *Homœopathy:* **Phosphorus**, **Hamamelis** or **Crotalus**
- *Herbs:* **Yarrow**
- *Essential oils:* **Cypress** or **Geranium** (inhaled)

Damage to cornea of the eye
- *Homœopathy:* **Merc. Corr.**
Topically in eye: **Euphrasia** tincture diluted – 2 drops in a eggcupful of boiled, cooled water

Combinations of the listed remedies may be used.

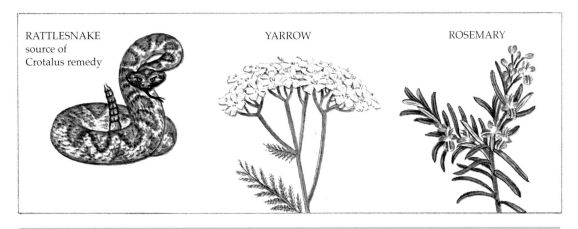

RATTLESNAKE
source of
Crotalus remedy

YARROW

ROSEMARY

Abscess

Abscess formation occurs in the case of penetrating wounds where there is deep infection or even a foreign body, such as a black thorn. The principle of treatment is the same, whether it be in the foot or elsewhere in the body. The abscess is the body's attempt to isolate and eliminate the infection and dead material and every effort should be made to encourage its formation and eventual rupture.

In the case of abscess in the foot, it is imperative to clear away the horn from the site of entry to allow proper drainage through the otherwise impenetrable material. A farrier will do this.

Foment the area by bathing in warm strong, salty water or strong Epsom salts solution.

A poultice can be applied, either soaked bread, soaked bran or proprietary starch or kaolin. Dried magnesium sulphate mixed with glycerine is also an extremely effective poultice. Do not over-poultice.

- *Homœopathy:* **Hepar sulph**. in early stages, three or four times daily; **Silica** in later stages, once daily, to resolve the abscess or to promote abscessation if it is inadequate; **Merc. sol.** may be of more help in cases of dental abscess
- *Herbs:* **Comfrey** leaves or **Slippery Elm** make a very good poultice. **Echinacea** internally
- *Essential oils:* **Bergamot** (local application)
- *Tissue salts:* **Silica**

(NB: Use of antibiotics may counteract the effect of natural remedies in this condition since they tend to delay abscessation.)

Allergy (including Urticaria)

See also **Cough.**

If a horse comes out in a rash of skin swellings, which can be circular or horseshoe-shaped, then there is usually an allergic reaction occurring. This may be due to a dietary factor or even to sudden changes in the bowel bacteria.

The condition can be very distressing and can cause facial swelling.

- *Homœopathy:* **Apis mel.** if more comfortable with cold applications; **Urtica** if more comfortable with warm applications
- *Herbs:* **Burdock**, **Cleavers** and **Dandelion**.
- *Tissue salts:* **Nat. Sulph.**

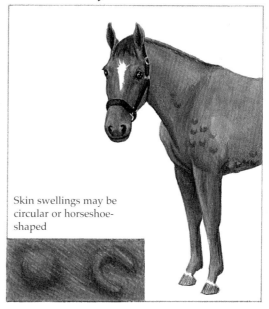

Skin swellings may be circular or horseshoe-shaped

Arthritis

Arthritis literally means 'inflammation of the joint' and is a general term covering anything from sprains (see page 11) to sesamoiditis. In most cases, proper regular therapeutic exercise routines should be adopted, integral with medical therapy. **Good nutrition is vital.** Conditions covered by these remedies are: arthritis of the knee, hip, shoulder, stifle, hocks (spavins), fetlocks, sesamoids, ringbone, etc. Foot problems are covered on pages 17-18. Incorrect saddling can be a major long-term cause of arthritic problems, due to the resultant wrong movement of the limbs. Ensure, therefore, that the saddle is correct and see also Back Problems (page 14).

- *Homœopathy:* **Rhus tox.** if the lameness is worse in cold, damp weather. The horse will 'limber up', will improve for stretching and enjoys rubbing of the joints. **Ruta**, similar but is effective where overstrain is the cause. Weight is shifted rapidly from one limb to another and there is less enjoyment of pressure. **Bryonia** if the lameness is improved for rest and if the horse is unwilling to move. The joint is often hot and painful. **Hekla lava** if there is prominent bone development at the joint
- *Herbs:* Useful herbs are **Comfrey**, **Devil's Claw**, **Burdock**, **Cleavers**, **Dandelion** and **Nettles**
- *Tissue salts:* **Ferr. phos.** or **Mag. phos.**, where there is muscle spasm. **Calc. phos.** and **Nat. phos.**, where there is stiffness. **Nat. mur.** where there is creaking in the joints
- *Essential oils:* A massage of **Camomile**, **Lavender** and **Hyssop** can be a very useful adjunct

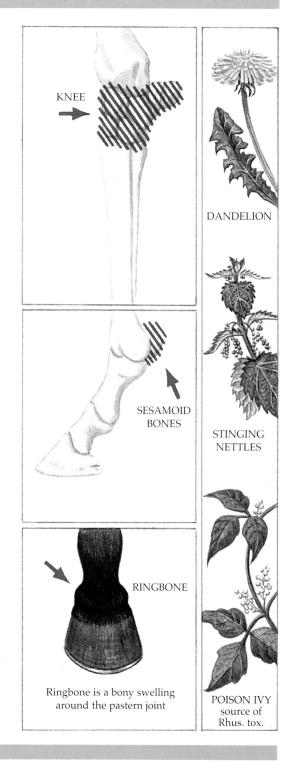

KNEE

DANDELION

SESAMOID BONES

STINGING NETTLES

RINGBONE

Ringbone is a bony swelling around the pastern joint

POISON IVY source of Rhus. tox.

Back Problems

Back problems constitute a very important and serious part of horse care and therapy.

Riding style, saddling and exercise routines all impinge very strongly on the integrity of the spine, as also do shoeing and dental alignment and function.

Apart from professional manipulation by a bona fide, properly qualified practitioner, therapies which may prove useful are:

- *Homœopathy:* **Rhus tox.**, **Ruta grav.**, **Arnica** or all three combined
- *Herbs:* **Comfrey**
- *Essential oils:* Massages of **Lavender**, **Rosemary**, **Eucalyptus** and **Hyssop**
- *Tissue salts:* **Mag. phos.**, **Nat. phos.**, **Kali. phos.** and **Nat. sulph.** combined

Other therapies

Laser and **ultrasound** therapy may also prove very useful as part of physiotherapy. These should only be used by well-qualified physiotherapists or veterinarians and used only as a supportive treatment to aid recovery.

Acupuncture, administered by an experienced veterinary surgeon, can prove very useful as part of an integrated therapeutic programme, but the back must be properly aligned first.

Massage can be carried out at home. The horse very quickly transmits his likes, dislikes and needs, so it is an easy and natural art to develop. Massage muscle masses (avoid bone); movements should generally be towards the heart to be compatible with circulation.

Magnets can be applied to painful areas.

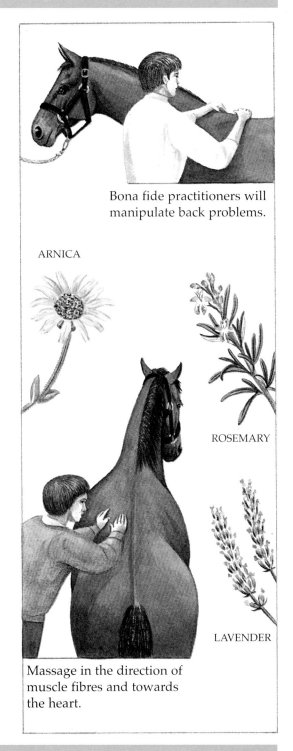

Bona fide practitioners will manipulate back problems.

ARNICA

ROSEMARY

LAVENDER

Massage in the direction of muscle fibres and towards the heart.

Colic

This is potentially a very dangerous condition so veterinary help and advice should be sought. However, in the first-aid situation before the veterinarian arrives, homoeopathic remedies can prove very helpful. Ensure teeth, diet and parasites are not a problem in order to try to prevent recurrence.

- *Homœopathy:* **Carbo. veg.** where gases are trapped and discomfort is noted; **Colocynth/Nux vom.** where cramping pains are a feature
- *Herbs:* **Angelica**, **Peppermint**, **Camomile** and **Valerian** will all help if the horse is still eating
- *Tissue salts:* **Mag. phos.**
- *Bach Flowers:* **Rescue Remedy** is a useful supportive treatment
- *Essential oils:* **Lavender** will help to calm the horse; **Camomile** and **Bergamot** will help to soothe spasms (by inhalation or on acupressure points)

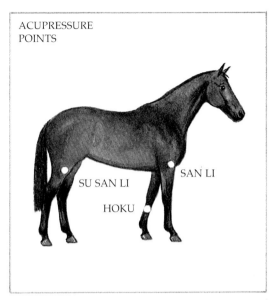

ACUPRESSURE POINTS

SAN LI
SU SAN LI
HOKU

Massage of these points will aid pain relief. Oils may be used.

Cough

There are a great many causes of coughs but two main categories are worth discussing: allergy and infection. The reason for distinguishing is so the appropriate preventive measures can be applied. Discuss these with your veterinary surgeon. Vaccination against influenza and other infectious respiratory diseases is not always desirable in every animal, nor is it always effective. However, competition regulations demand it at the time of publication.

- *Homœopathy:* **Drosera** – deep, harsh cough; **Bryonia** – cough worse for movement, horse is thirsty; **Nux vom.** – cough worse in the morning and in the fresh air; **Pulsatilla** – cough in a gentle horse, with greenish-yellow sputum, improved in fresh air; **Ipecacuanha** – spasmodic cough; **Arsenicum** – cough in a restless horse with thirst and a dry mouth
- *Herbs:* **Echinacea**, **Mullein** and **Sundew**
- *Tissue salts:* **Ferrum phos.** in the early stages; **Mag. phos.** in paroxysms of coughing; **Kali. sulph.** where discharges are yellowish and when the cough is better in the open air; **Silica** in cases of chronic cough
- *Essential oils:* **Eucalyptus**, **Cardamon**, **Jasmine** and **Peppermint** (by inhalation)

Diarrhœa

Clearly nutrition and grass quality must be checked. Parasites should also be assessed. Natural remedies can prove very useful. Persistent diarrhœa requires veterinary help.

- *Homœopathy:* **Arsenicum** if horse is thirsty, restless, tending to dehydration with a dry mouth; **Merc. sol.** where the mouth is wet and the horse is thirsty; **Nux vom.** if the horse has overeaten; **Colchicum** if the grass is too rich/wet; **China** after debilitating diarrhœa
- *Herbs:* **Agrimony**, **Comfrey**, **Cranesbill** and **Meadowsweet**
- *Tissue salts:* **Ferr. phos.** if sudden onset; **Nat. sulph.** – dark green dung; **Kali. phos.** – weakness with foul-smelling dung; **Calc. phos.** if there is also malnourishment
- *Essential oils:* **Camomile**, **Geranium**, **Peppermint** and **Sandalwood** (inhaled)

Discharges

Eye or nose discharges betray underlying ill-health and can be part of many other diseases. However, the most common cause is respiratory-type infection, or allergy. Ensure, in the case of eye discharges, that there is nothing in the eye (e.g. hay seed). Ensure hay is not of poor quality and is not dusty. Ensure proper ventilation in the stables and freedom from ammonia smells. Chronic sinus trouble will require more specialist natural medicine help, which should avoid surgery.

- *Homœopathy:* **Pulsatilla** – greenish yellow discharges, glands swollen, dullness, lack of thirst, worse in evenings; **Merc. sol.** – thirst with wet mouth, foul-smelling purulent discharges, glands swollen; **Hepar sulph.** – purulent discharge, high temperature, very painful swollen glands, tendency to abscessation; **Arsenicum** – watery corrosive discharges, restlessness; **Euphrasia** – use the tincture (diluted as on page 11) as a lotion in the eye in case of sore eyes with discharges; can also be used internally in homoeopathic potency
- *Herbs:* **Echinacea**, **Elder**, **Garlic**, **Mullein** and **Peppermint**
- *Tissue salts:* **Kali sulph.** if discharges are yellowish; **Kali mur.** – thick white discharges; **Nat. mur.** – low spirits, watery mucus; **Ferr. phos.** in early stages
- *Essential oils:* **Eucalyptus** or **Camphor** – may be used as an inhalant or applied to nostrils and can provide relief but do not use in conjunction with homoeopathic remedies; **Hyssop** may also help

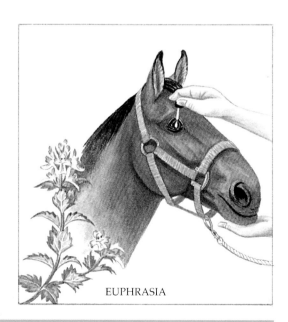

EUPHRASIA

Feet

The feet of your horse are of extreme importance and their health figures very importantly in a veterinary surgeon's daily work. Assuming that shoeing, management care and feeding are optimal, natural medicines which can help are:

Corns
- *Homœopathy:* **Arnica** internally. Bathe with **Hypericum and Calendula** lotion diluted 1 in 3
- *Herbs:* **Comfrey**
- *Essential oils:* Apply **Eucalyptus** oil

Cracks
- *Homœopathy:* **Graphites** – generally horse appears heavy and skin has poor healing ability; **Thuja** – the horse is averse to cold weather and has a tendency to warts
- *Herbs:* **Burdock, Chickweed, Comfrey** and **Nettles**

Poor hoof quality or growth
- *Homœopathy:* **Graphites, Silica**
- *Tissue salts:* **Silica**
- *Herbs:* **Burdock, Chickweed, Comfrey, Figwort** and **Nettles**

Pus in the foot
- *Homœopathy:* **Hepar sulph.** and **Ledum** in the early stages; **Silica** in later stages; Ensure adequate 'opening' of any wound. Your farrier or vet will most likely be needed. (See also Abscess page 12)

Sidebones and poor hoof flexibility
Too specialist for home treatment but herbal **Comfrey** and **Willow** can help

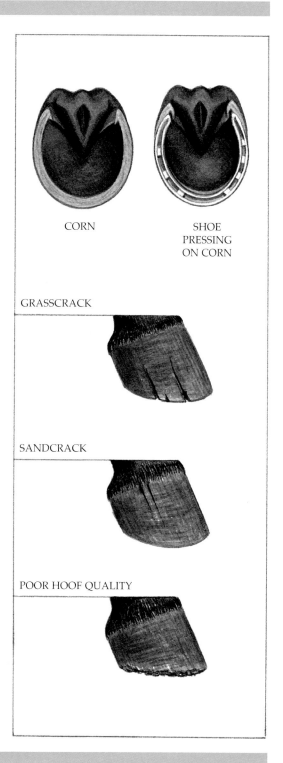

CORN

SHOE PRESSING ON CORN

GRASSCRACK

SANDCRACK

POOR HOOF QUALITY

Feet (continued)

Thrush
Regular thorough picking out of the feet will help to prevent this problem and careful trimming of the frog during farriery is essential.

- *Homœopathy:* **Hepar sulph.** internally should be used if the foot is sore and warm. In any case, **Hypericum and Calendula** lotion should be used externally, diluted about 1 in 3
- *Herbs:* **Echinacea**
- *Essential oils:* **Eucalyptus** oil is very useful in prevention, especially if pads are used on the foot for any reason

Navicular disease
Too specialist for home treatment but herbal **Comfrey** and **Willow** can prove very useful in relief of symptoms early on. Great success has been achieved in treating this disease, using a full holistic approach and natural medicine.

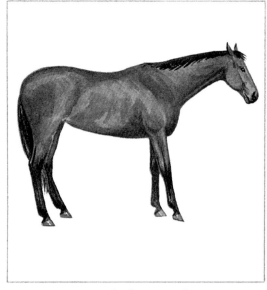

Typical stance of the horse with navicular disease. The horse 'points' his foreleg to obtain some relief.

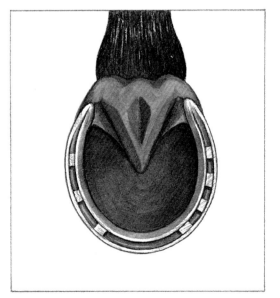

A well-shod foot, allowing flexibility of heel.

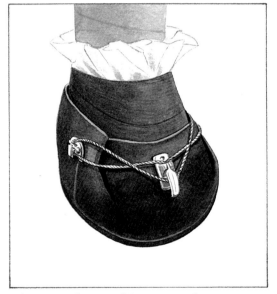

If you need to poultice, say to draw an abscess, a purpose-made protective boot will help to keep the dressing in place.

Laminitis

This is potentially a very serious condition which will most likely require specialist veterinary help in the selection of natural remedies and appropriate management. Nutrition is, of course, very important. Prevent access to grass (especially fertilised or 'improved' grassland), reduce concentrate intake and feed hard roughage in the first instance. Avoid feeds containing any added molasses or 'by-products of sugar production'.

Specialist farriery is a useful adjunct to treatment and, in severe cases, is essential. When the hooves are deformed by chronic laminitis and the pedal bone has moved, this is usually (but often incorrectly) assumed to be permanent and disabling. If at all possible, avoid heroic surgery of any sort and rely on specialist veterinary homœopathy, herbs and good, basic but intensive farriery.

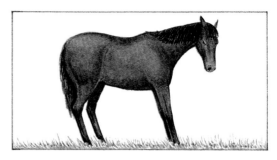

Characteristic stance of horse suffering from laminitis. (Swelling of the crest of the neck may be an early sign of the disease.)

In emergency first-aid situations use:
- *Homœopathy:* **Belladonna**
- *Bach Flowers:* **Rescue Remedy**
- *Herbs:* **Willow** – when painful

To help heal deformities:
- *Herbs:* **Comfrey**

Mud Fever/Greasy Heel

This condition can be very troublesome and may be due to buttercup sensitivity, excess clover, muddy conditions in the field, harvest mites or Dermatophilus infection. In any of these cases, appropriate steps should be taken where possible, to reduce exposure to the cause.

- *Homœopathy:* **Graphites** – skin cracks and sticky discharges; **Graphites** ointment may also be helpful; **Arsenicum** – sore, hairless, itchy skin; **Hepar sulph.** – where swelling and pain are uppermost symptoms
- *Herbs:* Topical – **Chickweed, Golden Seal, Marigold;** internally – **Burdock Root, Cleavers, Figwort, Nettle**
- *Tissue salts:* **Kali sulph.**

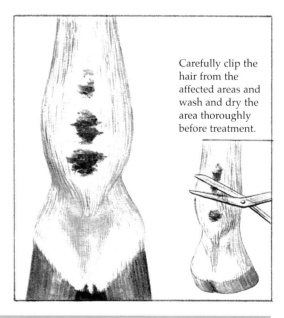

Carefully clip the hair from the affected areas and wash and dry the area thoroughly before treatment.

Nervousness and Excitability

This may be an inherent tendency in your horse but can be exacerbated by poor saddling, inappropriate stabling, incorrect feeding and handling. Sometimes it can be purely an exaggerated response to uncomfortable or unpleasant stimuli.

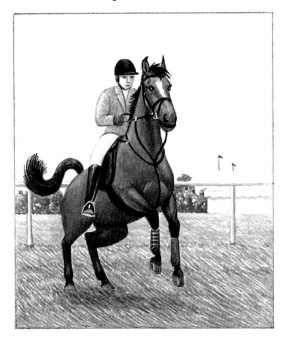

- *Homœopathy:* **Nux vom., Belladonna, Aconite, Stramonium**
- *Herbs:* **Hops, Skullcap** or **Valerian**
- *Essential oils:* **Basil** and **Lavender** inhalations will help
- *Tissue salts:* **Kali phos.**
- *Bach Flowers:* **Impatiens, Vervain, Scleranthus, Willow, Mimulus, Heather** or **Rock Rose**

Ringworm

Outbreaks of this can be very worrying and highly infectious. The condition usually responds well and rapidly to appropriate natural medicine. Only a few natural remedies will be mentioned. If they fail, more specialist veterinary help will be required to select others. Observe good hygiene principles, since the condition is infectious to human skin. A healthy skin and an untroubled mind are the best defences. For this, comfortable and unstressful conditions and a very healthy natural diet are vital, for horses and humans alike.

- *Homœopathy:* **Bacillinum**
- *Tissue salts:* **Kali sulph.**
- *Herbs:* **Echinacea, Cleavers** and **Yellow Dock**
- *Essential oils:* **Geranium** and **Peppermint** (by inhalation)

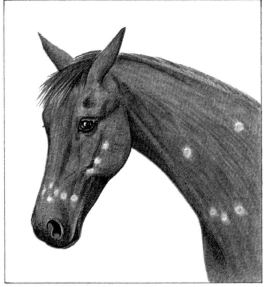

Hair loss in patches, sometimes weeping sores, unsightly scaly lesions and general unthriftiness and poor coat are the signs.

Saddle Sores

Incorrect saddling, ill-fitting rugs and poorly designed numnahs are causes. Quick and effective treatment, with immediate removal of the cause, is essential. If tack is so bad as to cause this condition, there is a serious welfare problem. Incorrect equipment should be discarded forthwith. Treatments which can be of help are:

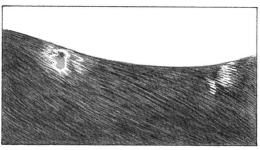

- *Homœopathy:* **Arnica** internally; **Hypericum** if pain is serious; **Arnica lotion** if skin is not broken; **Hypericum and Calendula** lotion, diluted 1 in 10, if skin is broken
- *Essential oils:* If skin is not broken apply **Lavender** and **Rosemary**
- *Herbs:* **Comfrey** internally and as an ointment
- *Tissue salts:* **Nat. mur.** and **Calc. sulph.**

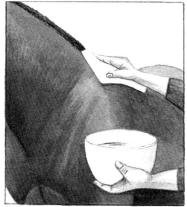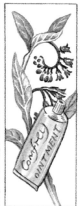

Splint

This annoying condition affects horses usually up to seven or eight years of age. It is an inflammation of one of the rudimentary digits alongside the cannon bones and usually affects the inside of the front limbs. It can be very painful but is rarely serious long-term. Permanent blemishes arise if the swelling does not reduce after the inflammation has subsided. In some cases the small bone may be fractured, demonstrable only by X-radiography, but treatment is similar.

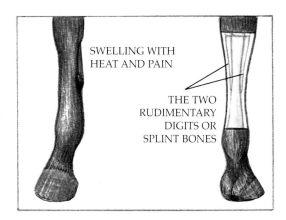

SWELLING WITH HEAT AND PAIN

THE TWO RUDIMENTARY DIGITS OR SPLINT BONES

- *Homœopathy:* **Arnica/Ruta** in early stages; **Symphytum/Hekla** in later stages
- *Herbs:* **Comfrey** internally or as an ointment and/or poultice
- *Essential oils:* A massage of **Eucalyptus**, **Lavender** and **Rosemary** may prove helpful
- *Tissue salts:* **Calc. phos., Nat. phos., Mag. phos.**
- *Magnets* can be applied to the area

Sprained Tendons, Ligaments and Muscles

The spraining or strain of tendons and ligaments can cause severe disabling of your horse. Riding should cease forthwith and regular gentle walking out exercise should be the order of the day, until healing is under way. There is a difference of opinion with regard to the advisability of box rest but, generally speaking, this author is against it as a rule, although rare special circumstances may demand its use. Factors predisposing to strain of tendons and ligaments are incorrect spinal and pelvic alignment, saddling, dentition, riding methods, exercise routines and shoeing.

Tendons and ligaments
- *Homœopathy:* **Arnica** in early stages, **Ruta** at all stages
- *Herbs:* **Comfrey**
- *Essential oils:* Massage of **Camomile**, **Camphor**, **Eucalyptus**, **Lavender** and **Rosemary**
- *Magnets* can be applied to damaged ligaments
- *Laser:* Regular therapy with laser may also prove very useful in the early stages

Sprained muscles/muscle injury
Broadly speaking, similar principles apply to muscle injury as to tendon injuries (above). Remedies to speed healing are:

- *Homœopathy:* **Rhus tox.** and **Arnica**
- *Herbs:* **Comfrey**
- *Tissue salts:* **Nat. phos.** and **Nat. sulph.**
- *Essential oils:* Massages of **Bergamot**, **Eucalyptus**, **Lavender** and **Rosemary**

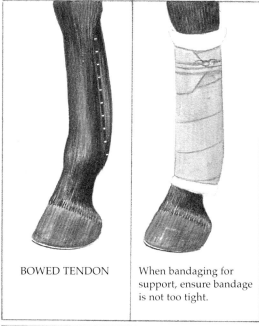

BOWED TENDON

When bandaging for support, ensure bandage is not too tight.

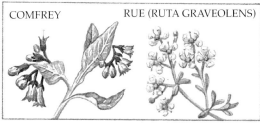

COMFREY   RUE (RUTA GRAVEOLENS)

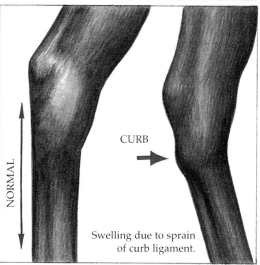

NORMAL

CURB

Swelling due to sprain of curb ligament.

Sweet Itch

This is a complex allergic-type condition affecting mostly native ponies and has a mixture of causes, each factor assuming different importance in each individual. Sunlight, midges and grass proteins all play a part. If the condition fails to respond to first aid home prescriptions, you are strongly advised to seek professional veterinary help in selecting further more appropriate natural remedies.

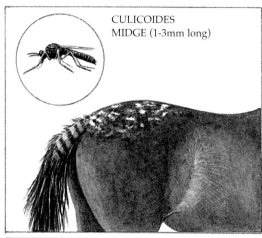

CULICOIDES MIDGE (1-3mm long)

- *Homœopathy:* **Graphites**; topical treatment with **Hypericum and Calendula** lotion diluted 1 in 10
- *Herbs:* **Cleavers, Echinacea, Nettles**
- *Tissue salts:* **Nat. mur., Kali. sulph.** and **Calc. fluor.**
- *Essential oils:* **Bergamot, Camomile, Geranium, Hyssop** and **Lavender**

Fly repellant oils - Cedarwood, Sandalwood, Pennyroyal, Catmint, Lemongrass and Lavender may be applied on a regular basis to reduce fly nuisance

Windgalls

This annoying swelling above the fetlock joints is often not at all disabling for your horse but betrays an underlying problem which should be addressed. The most common factors affecting the condition are diet, saddling and chronic, low-grade joint trauma. These should be scrutinised carefully, especially resorting to a totally natural diet, avoiding artificial additives and products and by-products of sugar production. Correct shoeing is essential too. The condition usually occurs during stabling; exercise is important for proper circulation and drainage.

- *Homœopathy:* **Apis mel., Ruta grav., Bryonia, Rhus tox.**
- *Herbs:* **Dandelion, Milk Thistle, Cleavers**
- *Tissue salts:* **Nat. mur.**
- *Essential oils:* Massage of **Eucalyptus, Juniper, Patchouli** and **Rosemary**

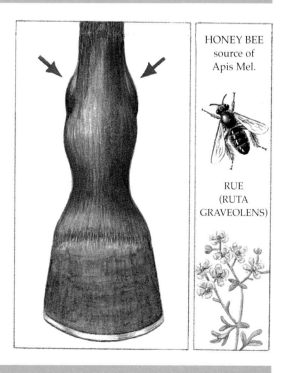

HONEY BEE source of Apis Mel.

RUE (RUTA GRAVEOLENS)

Guide to Dosing and Administration ▪▪

Always call in veterinary help if rapid improvement is not obtained.

Homœopathy

The 6c potency is the most widely available; 30c potency is an alternative, if available. As a general rule, twice a day dosing is acceptable, until improvement is noted. All preparations should be given by mouth, except the lotions. Dry preparations can be put in the mouth from a piece of folded paper or with a small piece of apple or bread; liquid preparations may be given direct from the dropper or in a small piece of apple. Combinations of homœopathic remedies can be used, but their effect is weakened. Do not touch the remedy.

Herbs

Herbs should generally be given as dry powder, or dried plant material. Tinctures are obtainable. Dosing should be once or twice daily, and the usual daily dose is about 20g, but does vary from herb to herb. By and large, avoid long-term use of herbs except under direction of a specialist veterinary surgeon. Always buy from a reputable source, taking care to ensure that labelling is correct and that no extravagant claims are made by the company. Herbs are usually given in the dry feed, e.g. with oats or a holistic feed mix.

Tissue salts

Give ten tablets twice daily until improvement is noted. Careful handling is essential, as per homœopathy.

Bach Flowers

These are obtained in liquid form and can be given direct in the mouth from the dropper, taking care not to contaminate the dropper with saliva or food. Twice daily dosing until improvement is noted; handle as per homœopathy.

Essential oils

These are very strong smelling and should be kept away from homœopathic medicines, tissue salts and Bach Flowers. Massages can be made up by putting a few drops with a carrier such as almond oil. This can be rubbed gently into the required area. Inhalations can be by steamer, burner (care required in a stable situation), or just by applying a drop near the nostril. They may also be applied next to an affected area or acupressure point, just putting a few drops on by finger pressure. Applications should be made twice daily until improvement is noted.

Magnets

A range of special magnets for local application is obtainable from veterinary surgeons or other outlets. Follow manufacturer's instructions or, failing that, apply the magnet to the desired area for a maximum of twelve hours in a day. If there is resultant heat or swelling, do not reapply until that has subsided. Cease treatment when the problem has improved sufficiently.